When the Grid Goes Down

Disaster Preparations and Survival Gear for Making Your Home Self-Reliant

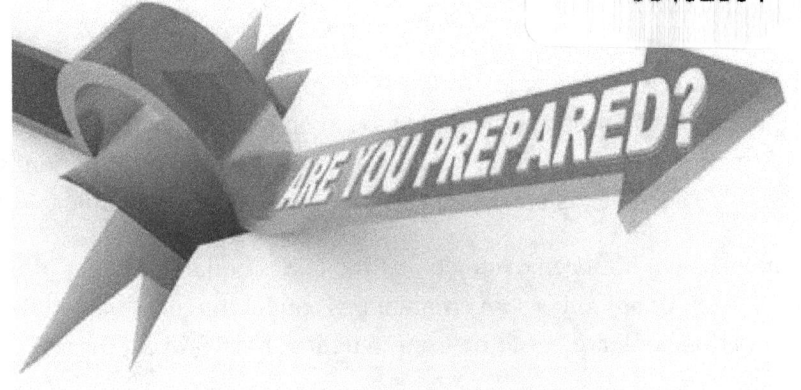

Prepping and Survival Series

M. Usman

Mendon Cottage Books

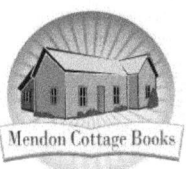

JD-Biz Publishing

Disclaimer

The information is this book is provided for informational purposes only. It is not intended to be used and medical advice or a substitute for proper medical treatment by a qualified health care provider. The information is believed to be accurate as presented based on research by the author.

The contents have not been evaluated by the U.S. Food and Drug Administration or any other Government or Health Organization and the contents in this book are not to be used to treat cure or prevent disease.

The author or publisher is not responsible for the use or safety of any diet, procedure or treatment mentioned in this book. The author or publisher is not responsible for errors or omissions that may exist.

Warning

The Book is for informational purposes only and before taking on any diet, treatment or medical procedure, it is recommended to consult with your primary health care provider.

Our books are available at
1. Amazon.com
2. Barnes and Noble
3. Itunes
4. Kobo
5. Smashwords
6. Google Play Books

Table of Contents

Preface

We will begin this book by providing you with the basics, such as the disaster supply kits. You have to be prepared for everything before any disastrous event takes place, because that is the only key to fighting off any mishaps that may occur. We not only give you the basic instructions, but will also supply you with the most important supply off all, the list of all the relevant objects you need. Now, a lot of these things are generally found in any common household, but we provide you with all other extra things that need to be there as well. We will follow it up with the advice of storing all important documents and what kind of documents are the important ones.

Disaster tools are followed by another key section, which is hygiene. When the grid goes down the usual setup of your life alters for a great amount of time, and the mechanisms that we normally rely upon are in disarray. Hence, we give you a list of essentials to make sure that your hygiene remains in good condition, because that will directly impact your health. Furthermore, that will potentially create problems for you in an already tough situation. In this section, we cover the basics all the way to creating a makeshift toilet.

The next section brings us to the issue of food. Here we give you all the do's and don'ts regarding food supplies. We tell you what foods you have to rely upon and those that you should avoid and keep at bay. Water, although more key in importance, comes after food in our book and after explaining its relevance, we will tell you all the different ways in which you can purify unclean sources for use. We follow it up with general advice with what steps to take during and after the blackout and sum it all up in a conclusion for you.

Read the book and follow it up with all the advice that we present to you. Remember: the key to prevention from any disaster is preparedness. We have done our part now it's your turn!

Chapter 1 - Introduction

The mere thought of a scenario where your grid goes down can be downright scary and troublesome for you. Fortunately this sort of situation doesn't happen too often and only an incident of a natural disaster can bring about such a calamity with it. However, we always need to be prepared for every scenario and these are extreme situations that require diligent preparation, a calm sense of mind, and the ability to know all the relevant steps that one has to take. Don't worry, as we are here for you for the exact same steps. We plan, through this book as a medium, to convey all the relevant details that will equip you with everything you need to know on how to fight this off.

1.1 Assemble a Disaster Supplies Kit

Having a disaster supply kit is always going to be the item of the foremost importance for you. These events are unfortunately almost always unforeseen and to be prepared for the unknown, you have to plan out for the worst, in order to be prepared at your best capability. Areas that are more prone to natural disasters have a higher risk of facing grid emergency situations. Hence, they should be even more alert and active in such planning. This is basically what this section will help in providing; listing out items, and picking the ones that are most important so that you do not miss anything of dire relevance in your hurry. One thing which has to be taken into account is that in all such preparations, the involvement of children is of absolute importance. This is so that they can also pitch in with practice and training and be aware of all the supplies and their locations in the situation of the grid failure.

1.2 Prepare Your Kit

Important Tips

- A kit in your car will come in handy. There are two advantages of this, with the first being that if the calamity strikes when you are away from home, you will not need to panic, as a smaller scale of a kit will be with you. Secondly when you face a grid failure you will have an additional back up supply of emergency items that may come in handy.

- Items have to be protected and not only stored in all such scenarios. Depending on what caused the grid failure, you will be most likely facing different scenarios. In case it was floods that hit you, then air tight plastic bags are very important to protect your equipment and other commodities.

- All the supplies have to be refreshed and the stocks should be replenished at least every six months.

- Drugs and prescriptions should be stocked up timely and with the help of your local pharmacist.

1.3 Disaster Supplies Kit Basics

The following list is a pretty basic list for you to check in your stores. This gives you a vague idea of everything that you need to gather.

- Flashlight

- Signal flare

- Extra batteries

- Supply of prescription medications

- First aid kit

- An extra set of car keys

- Personal identification

- A portable, battery-powered radio

- Matches in a waterproof container

- Cash

- Credit card

- Map of the area

1.4 Disaster Supplies Kit Basics

- Water will become an issue, so keep at least three gallons of water for each person stored. The details for that will be provided to you later on in this book.

- Cooking food is not going to be very easy for you therefore it is better if you keep a store of non-perishable food items that may last for a few days.

- Blankets

- Sleeping bags

- Important disaster tools and accessories: this is a very crucial section. Some of the objects that you may need to bear in mind can come extremely handy like pencil, paper, and threads and needles. Smaller packages or canisters may be used for items like a compass, plastic sheets, etc.

- Sanitation and hygiene items: this is going to become one of the major issues to be tackled when the grid goes out. The damages associated with the failure of grid include the possibility of lack of availability of water for sanitation and hygiene purposes. This will be catered to in a separate section as well, but you need to keep a mass storage of disinfectants, towels, and toilet paper to be safe.

Chapter 2 - First aid supply

The first aid supply section needs our special attention. Therefore, we provide you with a precise breakdown for all the items that you need to incorporate into the fit aid help box. Not only medications are required here, but there are several other important materials that you will need to incorporate in mediations or hygienic purposes.

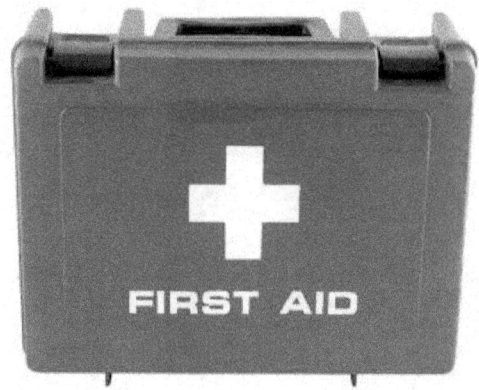

- Antibiotic ointment

- Eye drops

- Insect repellent

- Skin disinfectant spray

- Cold/Cough medicine

- Diarrheal medication

- Ear and nose drops

- Hydrogen peroxide

- Children's aspirin

- Benadryl
- Spare prescriptions
- Old pairs of eyeglasses

2.1 Drugs

- Eye drops
- Diarrheal medicine
- Antibiotic ointment
- Aspirin and non-aspirin tablets
- Hydrogen peroxide
- Prescriptions
- Wrapped alcohol swabs

2.2 Dressings

- Ace bandages
- Bandage strips
- Rolled gauze
- Cotton-tipped swabs
- Adhesive tape roll

2.3 Other First Aid Supplies

- Thermometer
- First aid book
- Paper cups
- Sunscreen

- Pocket knife

- Safety pins

- Tweezers

- Tissues

- Scissors

- Small plastic bags

- Sanitary napkins

- Needle and thread

- Bar soap

- Instant cold packs for sprains

- Splinting materials

2.4 Survival Kit for Your Home

- Screwdriver

- Adjustable wrench

- Ropes

- Hammer

- Axe, broom and a shovel

- Plastic sheeting and tape

- Pliers

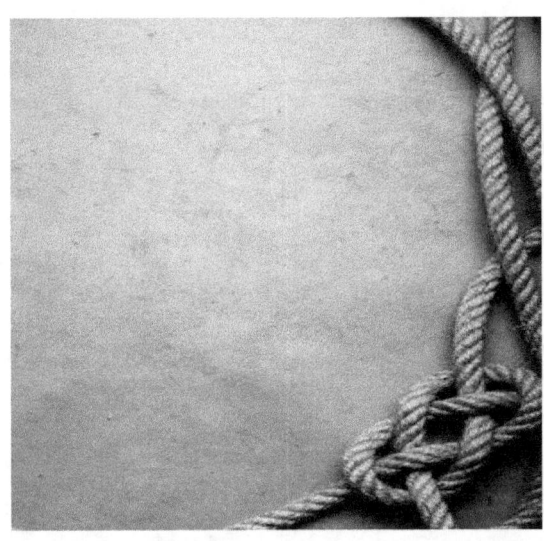

2.5 Items for safety and comfort

- Tent

- Candles

- Gloves

- Garden hose

- Waterproof matches

- Flashlight

- Blankets or sleeping bags

- Change of clothing

- Fire extinguisher

- Cash

- Portable radio

- Knife

- Food and water for pets

- Strong shoes

- Essential medications and eyeglasses

- Toilet tissue

2.6 Survival Kit for Your Automobile

- Change of clothes

- Food

- Jumper cables

- Whistle for signaling

- Flashlight

- Toilet tissue

- Blankets

- Gloves

- Paper and pencils

- Fire extinguisher

- Compass

- Battery-type flasher

- Light sticks

- Bottled water

- Local maps

- Duct tape

- Coins for telephone calls

- Reflector

- Prescription medicines

- Battery-operated radio

- Small mirror for signaling

- Ropes

- First aid kit and manual

2.7 Important Documents

There are a few personalized documents that are very important for various factors. Now, in order to make sure that you obtain them with comfort, you need to ensure that all the documentation has been safely stored in easily accessible areas. Preplanning, as we've repeatedly asked of you, is the key to all locked doors. The following is a list that incorporates almost all of the necessary documentation.

- Immunization records

- Social security cards

- Contracts

- Bank account numbers

- Stocks and bonds

- Insurance policies

- Family records (birth, marriage, death certificates)

- Inventory of valuable household goods

- Will

- Passports

- Credit card account numbers

- Important telephone number

2.8 Disaster Tools

Tools are always a life saver and their aid can be required at any moment in time. In the extremely short time period, there will be a panic for anything really so therefore if we can equip ourselves with all necessary items, the panic mode can be reduced fairly

- Bleach
- Battery operated radio
- Multipurpose tool
- Trash bags
- Wrench to shut off gas
- Tube tent
- Can opener
- Signal flare
- Waterproof matches
- Survival manual
- Floatation device
- Fire extinguisher
- Pliers
- Propane stove
- Plastic cups and plates
- Whistle

- Duct tape

- Extra cash

- Map

- Compass

Now it is quite clear that the matter of a grid failure is unforeseen, but you can always analyze the turn of events around you, if you are observant. The failure of a grid, as we initially explained, can be from occurrences of natural calamities or in the events of a terrorism activity. All you need to ensure is that you act on the matters that are solely in your hands and of what you are responsible. If you plan early and ensure the collection of the stated items timely and orderly, you can avoid the moments of panic and combat the grid failure with more bravado. Be ready for the worst and hope for the best.

Chapter 3 - Hygiene

During normal life routines keeping hygiene is not really much of an issue that you may consider, but it all changes when the grid goes down. The supplies are now limited and your trusted companion, the water supply, is not something that may be relied upon now. Lack of sanitation has been attributed to hundreds of deaths in the grid failure situations. In such scenarios, keeping control of your environment in the matters of sanitation becomes even more crucial. Consider for an instance that the failure of the grid has been brought about by the floods in such circumstances the spread of diseases are going to increase and the hygienic environment becomes an all important factor to be controlled.

3.1 To Build a Makeshift Toilet

Using your natural commodes for toilet purposes may not be a very good idea, as there will be a water shortage to clean up the created waste. A makeshift toilet in such scenarios will make it easier for you to dispose of the waste in a more hygienic and convenient way. The process is very simple and all you need to do is to wrap a garbage bag over a bucket and use that as a makeshift toilet. The disposal of the waste is hence made easier. Use disinfectants to make sure that the spread of germs is contained and cleanliness is ensured. Bury the waste properly or dispose of it in a proper area.

The rest of the sanitation items are not really an issue. The basic problem at that time would of course be their availability to you. There are ready made kits for this purpose available in the markets, for your convenience, so you can buy them beforehand (clearly you can't delay that). The other obvious thing is to collect them separately and yes that is exactly what we are going to do for you now. The following are a few select necessary items that you'll need.

Toilet Paper: This is something you seriously need a little extra of, even more than usual. The fact remains that toilet paper is one of the most crucial items on your sanitation list. At the time of aid, any paper will do the task, but it would be better to avoid an uncomfortable situation as water usage is especially going to be very restrictive. In the scenarios of floods, there might also be stomach diseases urging you to use the toilet more often.

Oral Hygiene: Extra toothbrushes can always come in handy. Oral hygiene is one of the most important ones for your health. A well maintained oral health system can protect you from most diseases.

Deodorants & Air fresheners: Not only personalized smells are to be made better in every situation, but how your surroundings smell also changes your mood and temper. The comfort levels can be enhanced and the sense of smell can ease up the situation for you.

Hair Supplies: Remember this is a survival scenario and not a fashion preparation, but still you can pack smaller amounts of such sanitation items. Shampoos, some combs, and hand sanitation lotions can always come in handy.

Bathing: Water is a commodity that you cannot afford to waste. Hence priority has to be given to utilizing the water for eating and drinking purposes as well as washing hands. Apart from all such activities, it is very important to take baths. The chance for you to have them is at close by fresh streams. Be careful though and always wear shoes to prevent infections and wounds. Always use biodegradable soaps and sanitizing lotions for washing purposes.

Designated Sanitation Area: Choosing the correct location for the disposal of waste is as important as any medication for a disease. The disposal place should be downhill and far away from any usable source of water. If the waste can be buried away that will be a very good attitude, as it will prevent infections. Otherwise disposal has to be made carefully and the garbage should only be thrown away unceremoniously. Keep the throwing area downwind from living areas too if you can help it. Let us now give you the proper methodology for burying your refuse.

Choose a location downhill, away from any springs, wells, and water supplies. Dig a hole at least twelve to eighteen inches deep and at least one hundred feet downhill. Always fill the pit with dirt after throwing down the waste.

Chapter 4 - Food

Living in the countryside can attract various animals; make sure that no food items that you waste get piled up. You should either burn or bury the food waste. Keep the water and your food covered, as contamination of food is something that you cannot really afford at this time. This is probably the best time to utilize your resources scarcely. Make only enough food to be consumed in one sitting and do not wash dinner plates with the water supply that is reserved to be drunk.

4.1 Food for survival:

When the grid goes down, everything becomes sort of stagnant. The panic starts to seep in, you do not know how long this will continue, and you are worried about your family and their survival. In this life, we have surrounded ourselves with this mechanization and have become so dependent on the energy sources to continue living our lives. We have become slaves to the energy sources and without them we fluster. This grid failure can be fought off, but the only thing that worries you are all problems that can be tackled such as, food, water, hygiene, and protecting your family. Don't worry, we shall cover them all. Let's start by walking you through some of the best survival foods which you need to stock up on in order to fight of one of the problems in your list.

MRE

Yes, that's quite the first thought by reading "MRE" isn't it, you will be wondering what kind of a special formula this is supposed to be. Well "MRE" is one of the most specialized foods invented by the military to be used in their strict survival training programs. Now bear in mind that these are" meals ready to eat" and have been introduced by the military for situations where food preparation is not possible. Keeping in view how expensive these are and how specialized they are, we do not recommend that you buy these in bulk, but keeping a few in your store can become a benefit for you.

Rice

Found to be a delicacy in some meals and a main component in others, rice is a main part of our everyday meal combinations. Keep a good amount of rice stored in your stock. You can get a ten pound bag of rice for around five dollars and this should at least be in your pantry at all times. High carbohydrates and loads of physical energy are what these important little grains can offer you. Another plus point is that it has a storage life of up to ten years.

Beans

Beans are without a doubt one of the best survival foods. Packed with proteins, they are fit to be consumed for around ten years given that they are kept in a sealed food grade bucket with a tiny amount of dried rice. Buy four to five pounds of this delicious power packed food every time you visit the grocery store and keep them stored in a cool and dark environment.

Cornmeal

Out of all the flours, one of the best in order to store is the cornmeal. Not only is it jammed with carbohydrates, but it also contains select oils that help in giving it a much longer life.

In the grid failure situation cornmeal becomes your best friend, as it is very easy to make a corn bread with a skillet or a solar oven. It has to be stored like beans with dried rice and a little salt. They are fit to be consumed within two years.

Lard

Yes I know if you are really healthy conscious lard does not come upon as a very appealing option. But, when you are considering survival food choices, lard has a fighting chance to fit in to your meal schedule. Now it has the necessary calories and also it is an excellent alternative to your cooking oil because of the process of hydrogenation. It is also to be stored in dark and cool places. The cellar or your basement is good options and it can be fit for consumption for around two years.

Salt

If you are looking for the savior of your survival foods, stop right here. Salt is the best and most useful of the survival food ingredients. The strongest quality that salt brings to the table apart from flavoring our every meal is that it can last forever.

Sugar

There are two kinds of sugar that you will need in your storage unit for survival foods; one is brown sugar and the other is the white sugar. Both provide you with the all the important flavors and necessary calories. If taken care of, they are fit to survive ten years. They are not an expensive commodity therefore buy extra as they are almost always under heavy usage.

Pasta

Now there is a household favorite. The list is getting tastier as we proceed. One of the best light weight foods for your diet is the pasta. Pasta, the extremely tasty and light weight food, is a great source of carbohydrates. Pasta doses not remain fit as long as rice, as around five years is their limit in good conditions. However, it does take up a lot more space in your food reserves than rice and beans so you should plan its buying wisely.

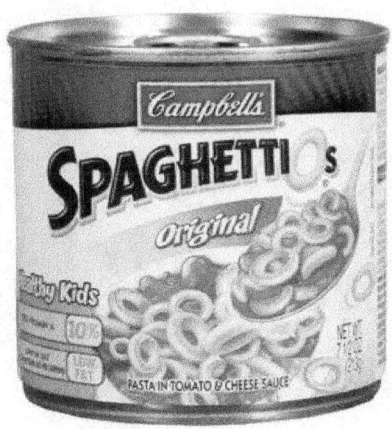

Peanut butter

Talking about light food, peanut butter has to cross your mind. It's a great treat to have with you, filled with protein and calories, and it can be a great companion.

Chapter 5 - Water

Water is the basic necessity for life. It is the utmost important factor for our continued survival in this world. Nothing can be more important than the availability of water for our everyday needs. The human body is made up of approximately sixty to eighty percent water. There is no way that a human body can perform its usual activities with the efficiency it possesses, without water. The variation in the task will of course lead to a difference in the intake requirement.

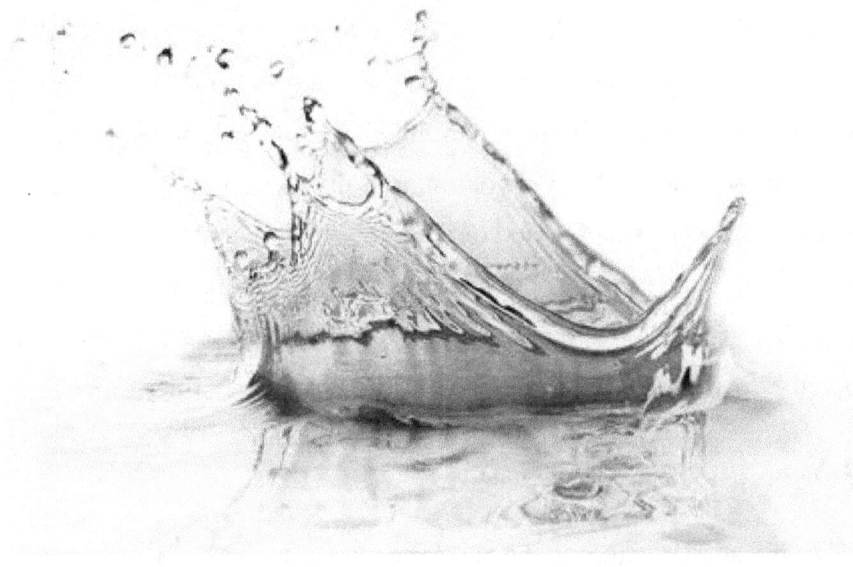

In the situation where the abundance of the water supply is an issue, we can take a few precautions to ensure that the amount of water that we have at our disposal is used to its maximum potential.

Firstly, we can ensure that the demands of our body can be restricted by some amounts. For that to happen, we have to cover any exposed skin to the sun. This will protect against sunburn and water losses through the damaged cells. In arm conditions, covered skin also helps in the reduction of evaporation of heat from the body. By doing all this, we are basically ensuring that the need to replace the bodily fluids is reduced.

Wearing loose clothes by the same argument is better than wearing those that are comparatively tighter. The tighter garments trap the air around the body hence insulating the body. The trapped area creates humidity and thus leads to more heating.

In taking water

You have to ensure that you only eat according to the water reserves that you have left. You need to have a moderate source of hydration otherwise eating far too much would only result in your body demanding way too much water than what you might currently have in your storage. Another very important thing to keep in your mind is that you should not swallow too much water in a small period of time. It is advised that you only drink when you feel really thirsty or dehydrated. The logic behind this advice is that the body is designed to process little quantities of water at a little time and that's why these breaks can help you out in water shortage times.

5.1 Ways to purify water

In case of water shortages in the pure water reserves, here are a few methodologies that you can use to turn the impure water into drinkable water sources.

By far the easiest way to cleanse water is to boil it. Be it campfire or open sun. Depending upon the severity of your situation, you can always do this process. Bring the water over a heat source and wait until you have bubbles appearing on the surface. Let the water boil for a sufficient time and always let the water cool down afterwards; do not be impatient.

A purification pump

Also known as a filtration pump, it can be used to purify water as well and make it drinkable. Any basic supply store has it available and you should stock it up before any disastrous situation occurs. The basic mechanism of this instrument is that it squeezes water through ceramic and charcoal areas of the filter and treats it with chemicals. Now with recent advancements in technologies there are some high technology water bottles also available in the market that do this process for you and all you have to do is enjoy a safe and clean supply of water.

Purification drops

These are also available with the name of purification tablets are also really useful sources of purification. The most commonly available purification tablet is iodine, but others are available in the market are under the names of potassium permanganate or chlorine. Note that do not put the exact alternative chemical directly, but go to a prescribed store for such purpose. Make sure that you give the chemical at least half an hour to treat the water supply before you decide to consume it. There are also powdered mixtures available in the markets that treat the taste of the water which may be deteriorated by the presence of the chemicals in the water. One important thing about this water is that it cannot be used indefinitely as water normally can be. This kind of water now has an expiry date, which normally lasts for one year, but there may be variations in that date. Do not place the tablets with your hands as they should not come into contact with them. Use a pair of tweezers for this purpose.

Another great new methodology is water purification straw. This can be used to clean up to one hundred and twenty gallons of water. Isn't that really helpful? You can acquire this from any supply store and it is easily accessible and easy to use.

This last method is to be used for emergency purposes only and we hope that you don't have to use it but hey, you have to learn.

Turning salt water or urine water into drinkable water

Yes it seems to be the least likely and pleasant source that you might want to drink, even after you have purified it. What you need to make this process work are a couple of containers with lids and a connecting metal rod. You have to place the container that has impure water in it, over the heat. Place the other container over a higher ground level. The process that follows is basic distillation. The water vapors from the impure container will follow along the rod into the pure container and there you have it, water is fit and ready to be consumed.

Chapter 6 - Blackouts

6.1 What to do during a blackout

• Always only use flashlights for all purposes. Never even think about using candles, as they pose a very serious risk of fire.

• Since you are out of electricity, you have to ensure that you keep your refrigerator doors locked, do not open and close them regularly. Let the cold be stored for the maximum amount of time.

• Be very careful regarding any spoilage of food items.

• Make sure that all major appliances are disconnected from the main power supply. Electricity may make a few appearances momentarily and there may be surges in voltages. This will prevent appliances from getting damaged.

- Make sure your generator is not connected to the main household supply; this will only waste the energy of the generator. Connect the generator only to the few relevant items that you require immediately.

- Always keep updated through the radio. Keep spare batteries always. This cannot be stressed enough.

- Also, leave one light always on so that you can monitor when your electricity gets back. Make sure you do not use the phone unnecessarily as it may come of great help in case of any further emergency.

- At this time, everyone will be in a panic mode. Make sure you remain calm and don't call 911 for UPDATES. This server should be kept for reporting relevant emergencies only.

- Use warm clothes for protection against the cold weather, but never burn charcoal for protection against the cold weather.

6.2 After the blackout

Do not feel the necessity to keep any food that is in doubt. Specifically, if any food has been exposed to forty degrees Fahrenheit, throw that away. Even if the food appears to be in a fine state and smells nice, if it has been exposed to such temperatures, then there is always a risk that it has been infected with bacteria. Some of them may not even be destroyed by cooking it further.

Conservation of energy is extremely important, so do whatever you can to ensure that you save as much as possible. Do not think that what you save will be insignificant, because every watt saved will, in the long run, be effective for the community and in effect the entire country. Small steps are necessary like using heavy appliances only during late nights or early mornings. When the temperatures are high, do not keep the air conditioner running when you aren't home. If you want to make sure that the room temperature is bearable before you come back ensure that you use a timer.

Chapter 7 - Conclusion

Go for green energy and make sure that you buy energy efficient products. Avoid standby losses from products like televisions and other electronic devices that remain plugged in. Remain calm during a disaster and do your bid for the community as well. If you and your family are safe, go out and about to look for anyone who might need your help. Helping others is what is expected of good natured people. Follow all that we have tried to convey and you will find yourself safely wading your way through the disaster. Remember that it is always key to mark your priorities, keep a cool head, protect your family, seek and save food and water, search for important disaster tools, protect important documents, and then spread out help in your society. Keep yourself and your family and then the community safe and give all the help that you can.

Author Bio

Muhammad Usman is a distinguished medical graduate of Allama Iqbal medical college (AIMC). He is a professional writer who has been in the field for more than 4 years. During this time he has produced 10,000+ articles, blogs and eBooks on various niches related to diseases, health, fitness, nutrition and well-being. He is a regular contributor to several journals related to medicine and surgery. He is the editor of several journals and newspapers.

Check out some of the other JD-Biz Publishing books

Gardening Series on Amazon

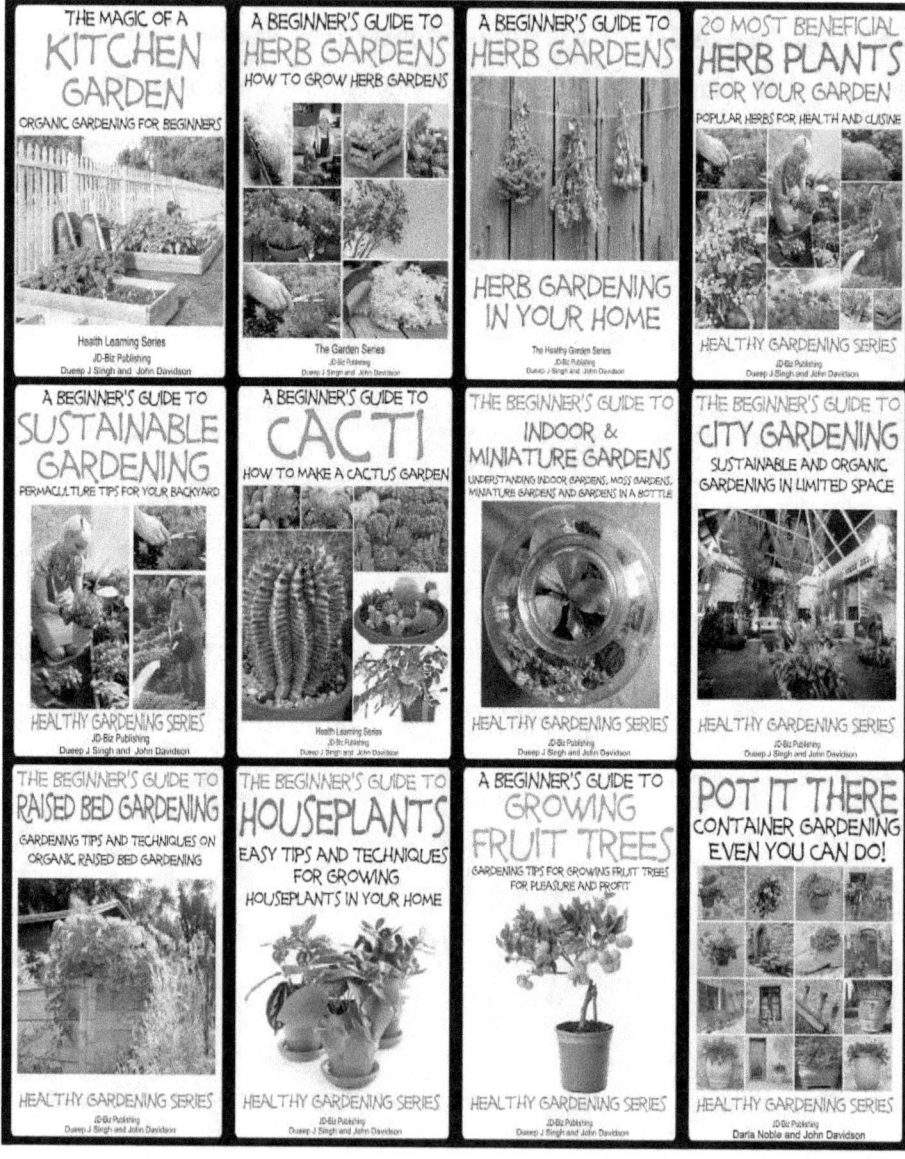

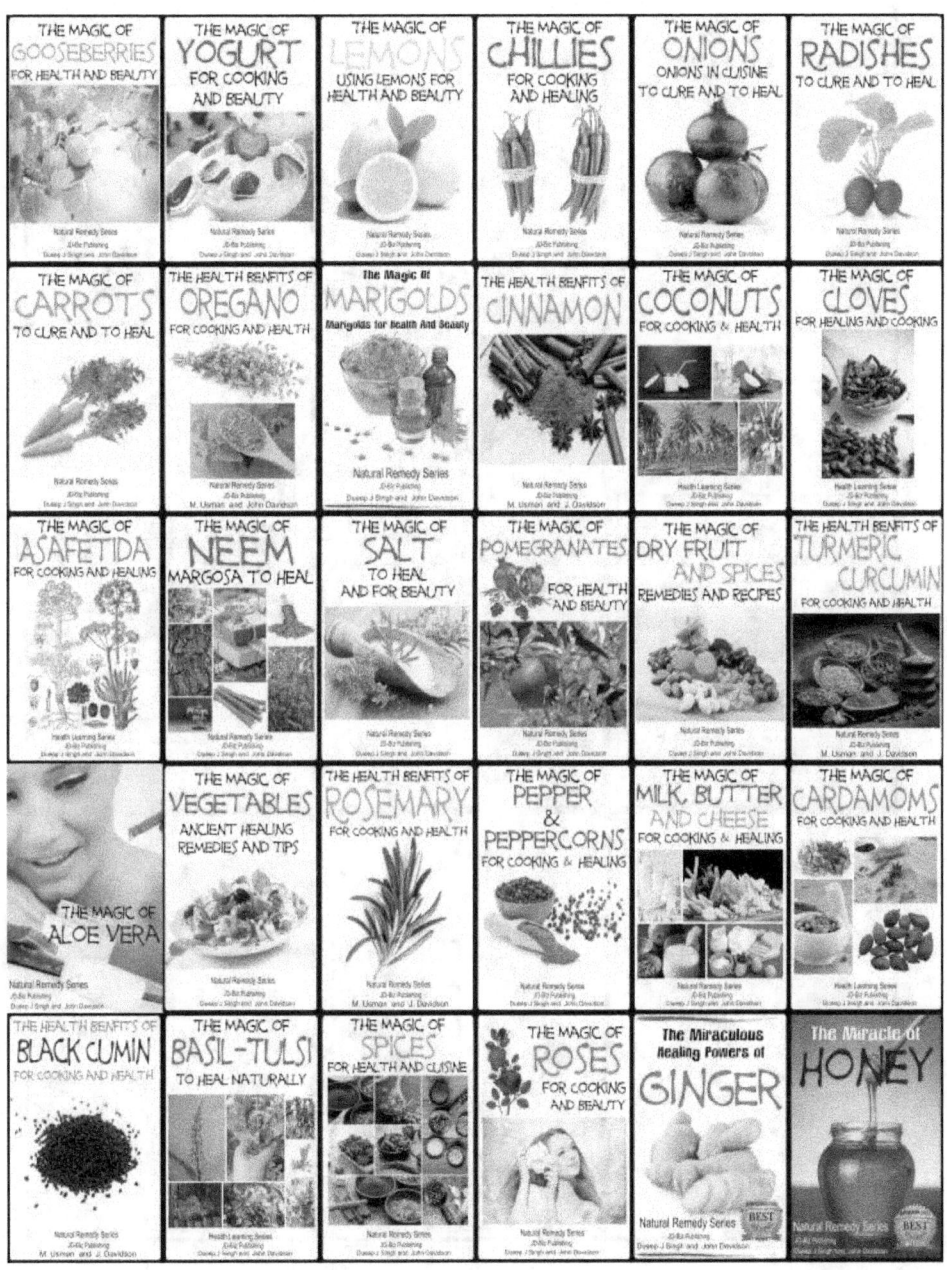

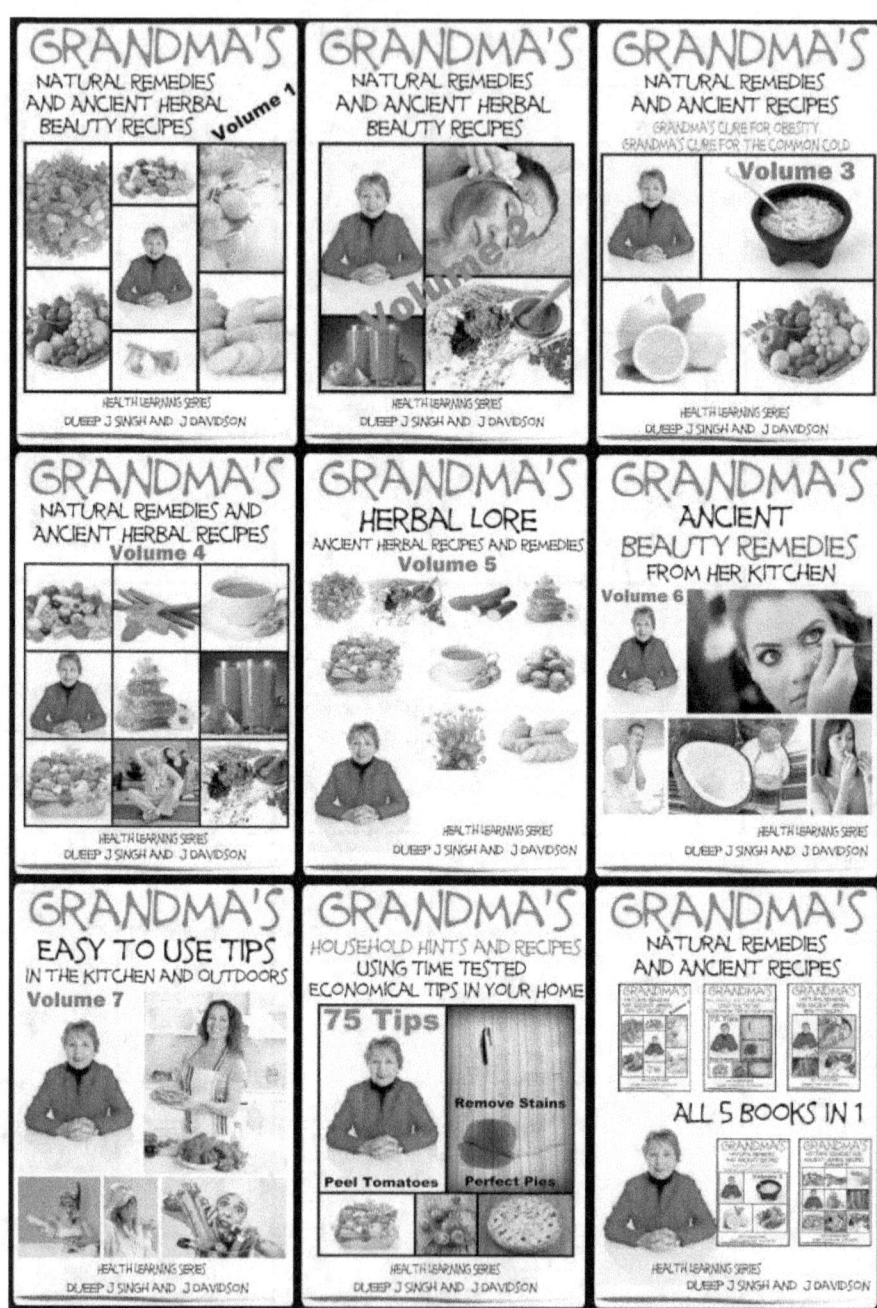

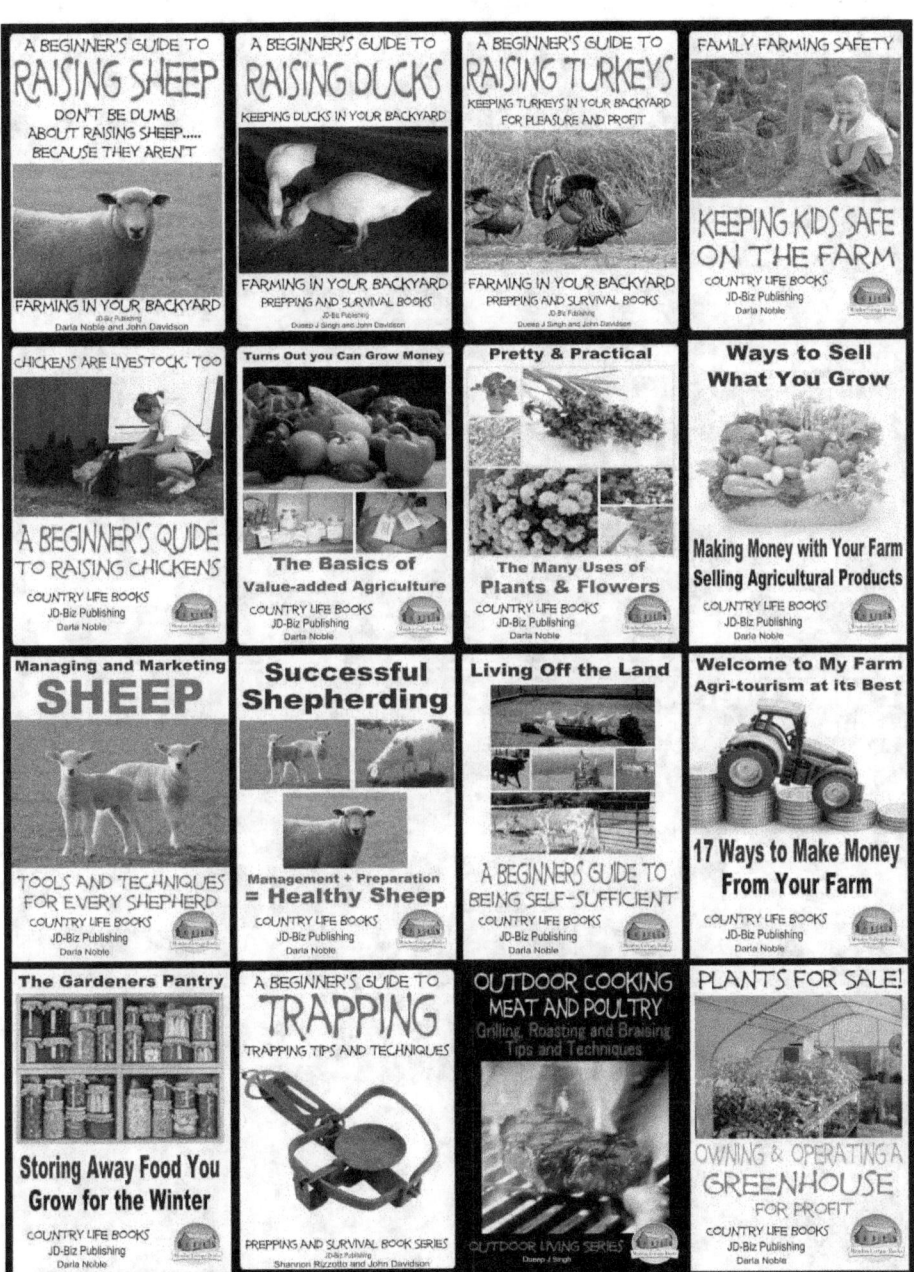

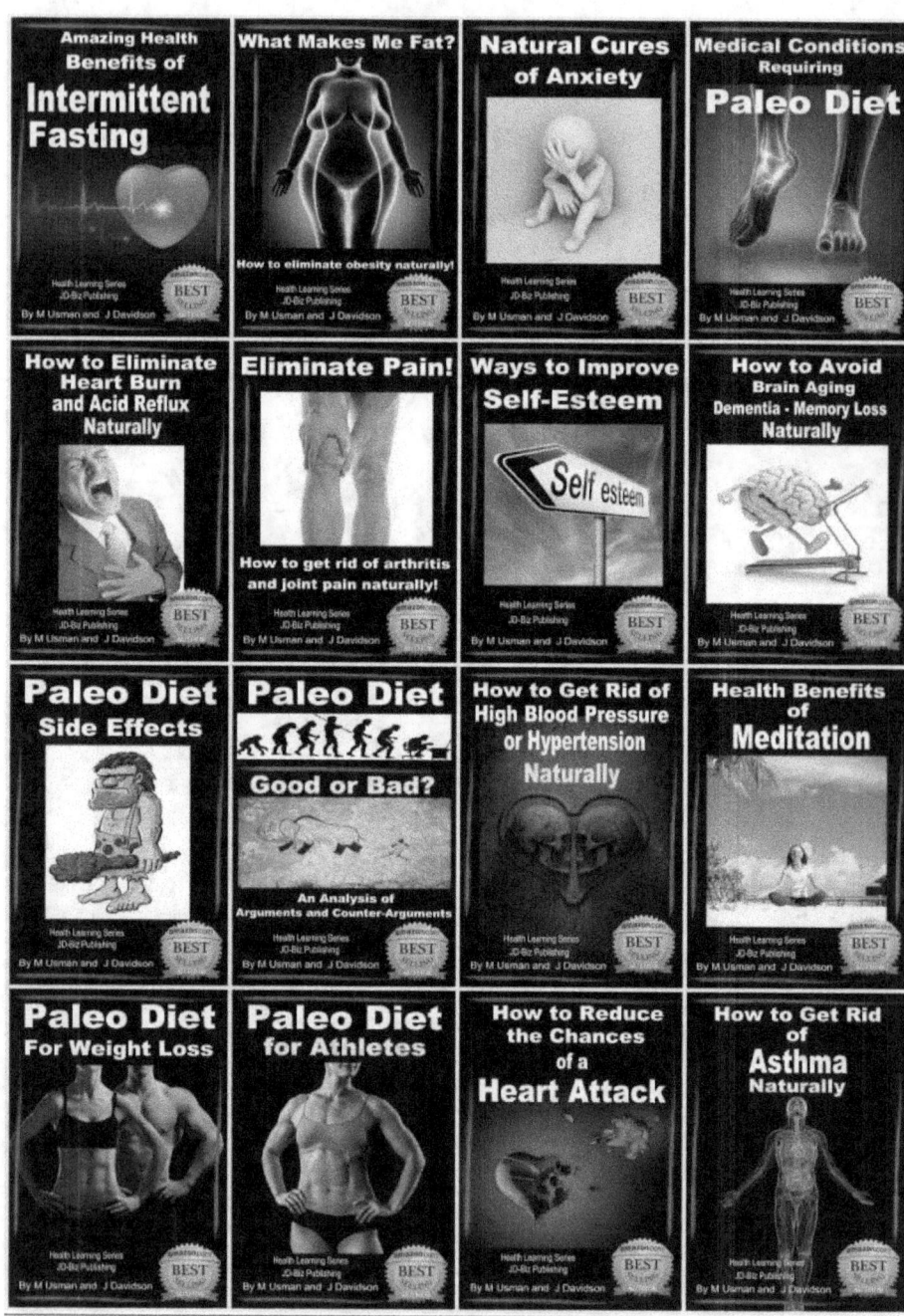

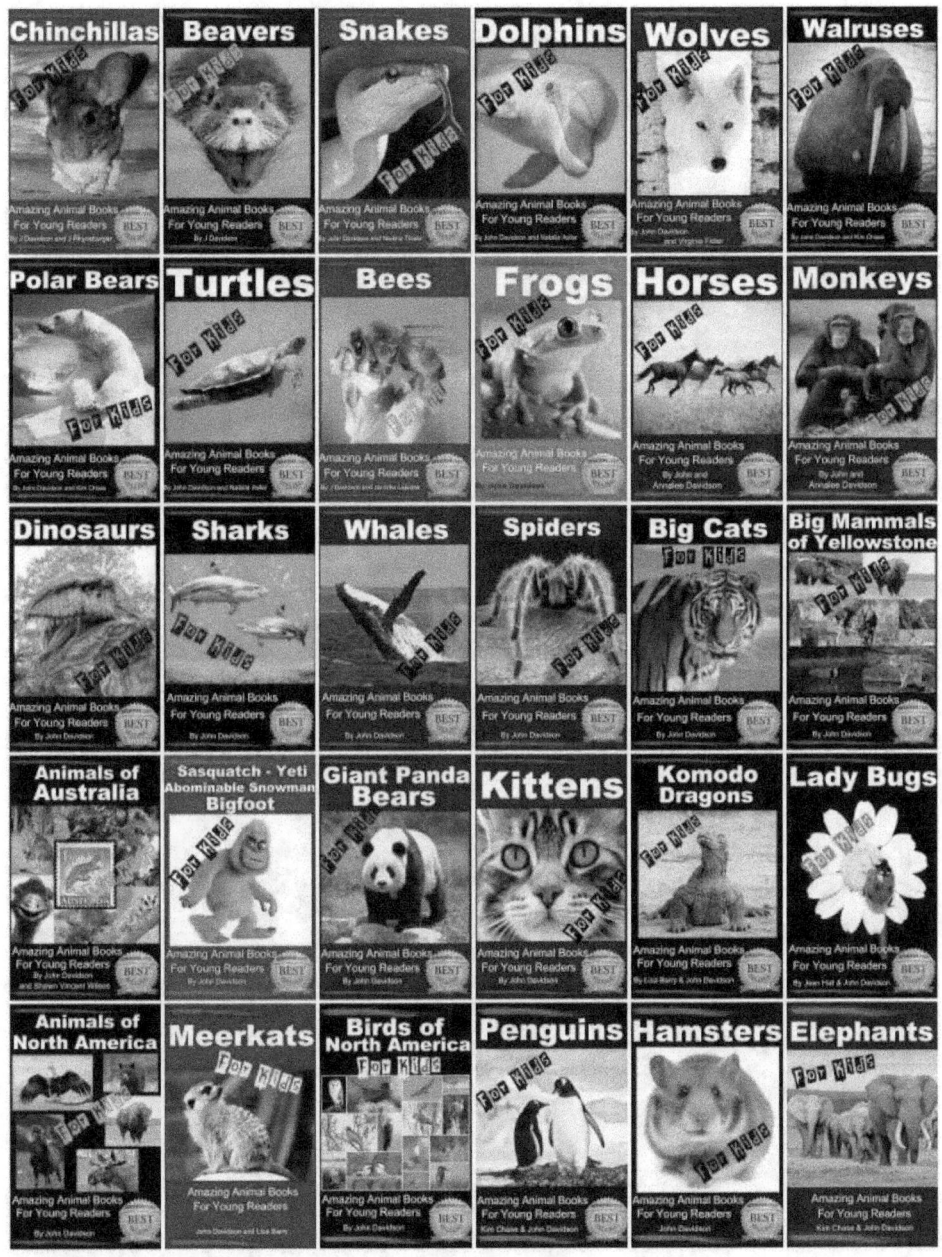

Learn To Draw Series

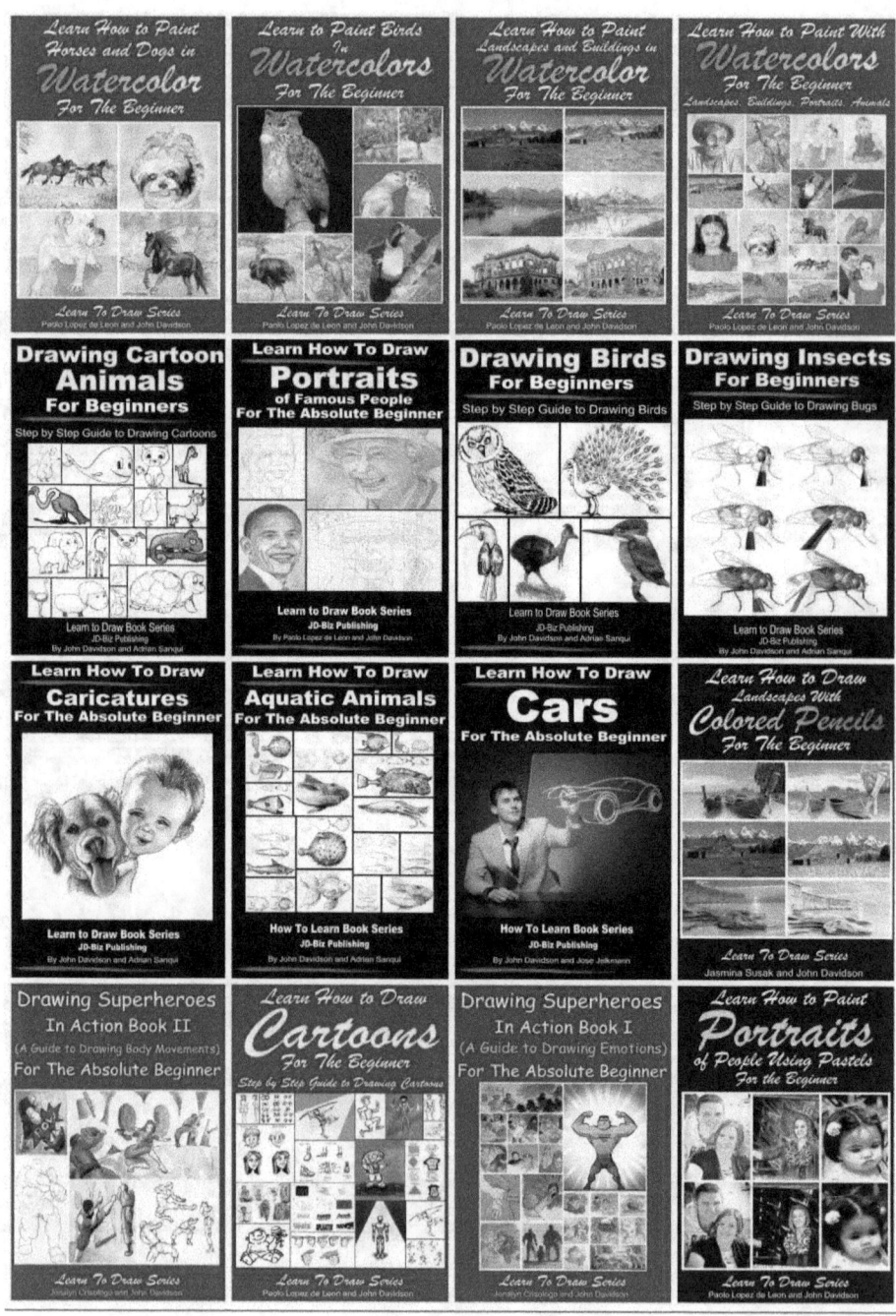

How to Build and Plan Books

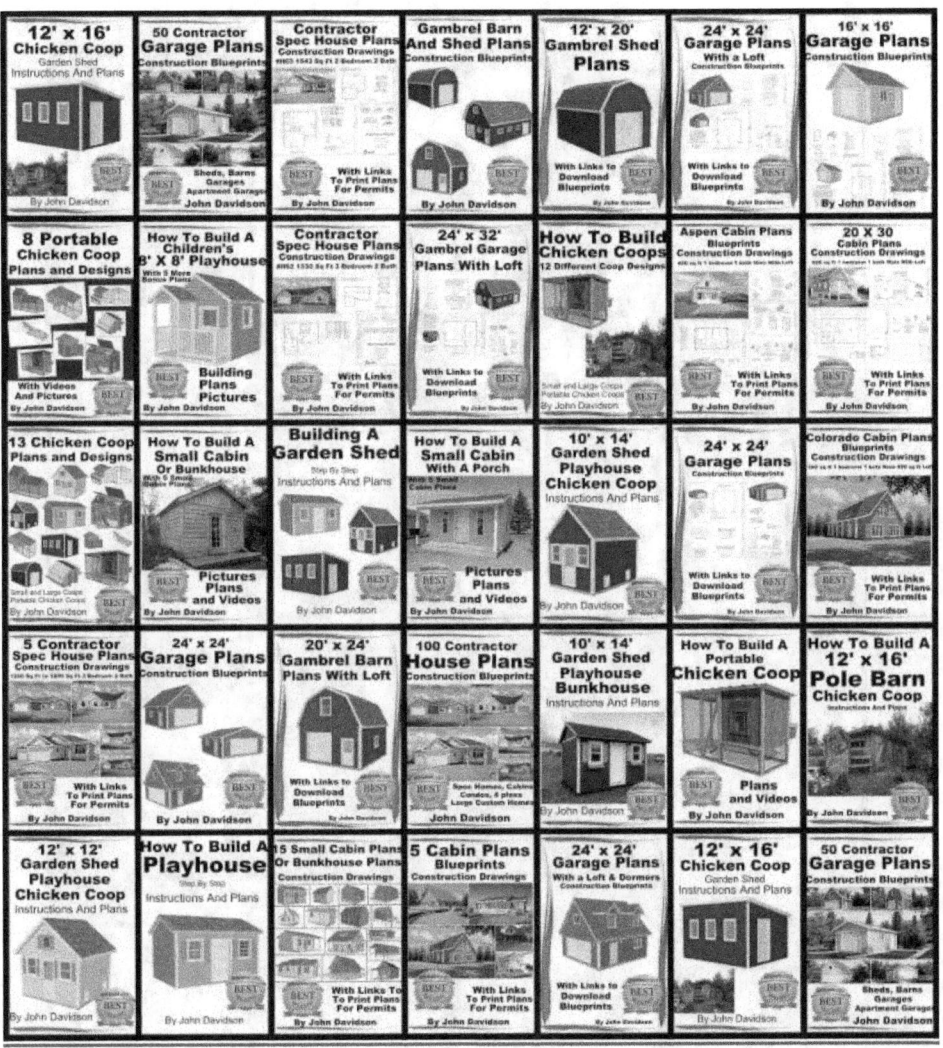

Entrepreneur Book Series

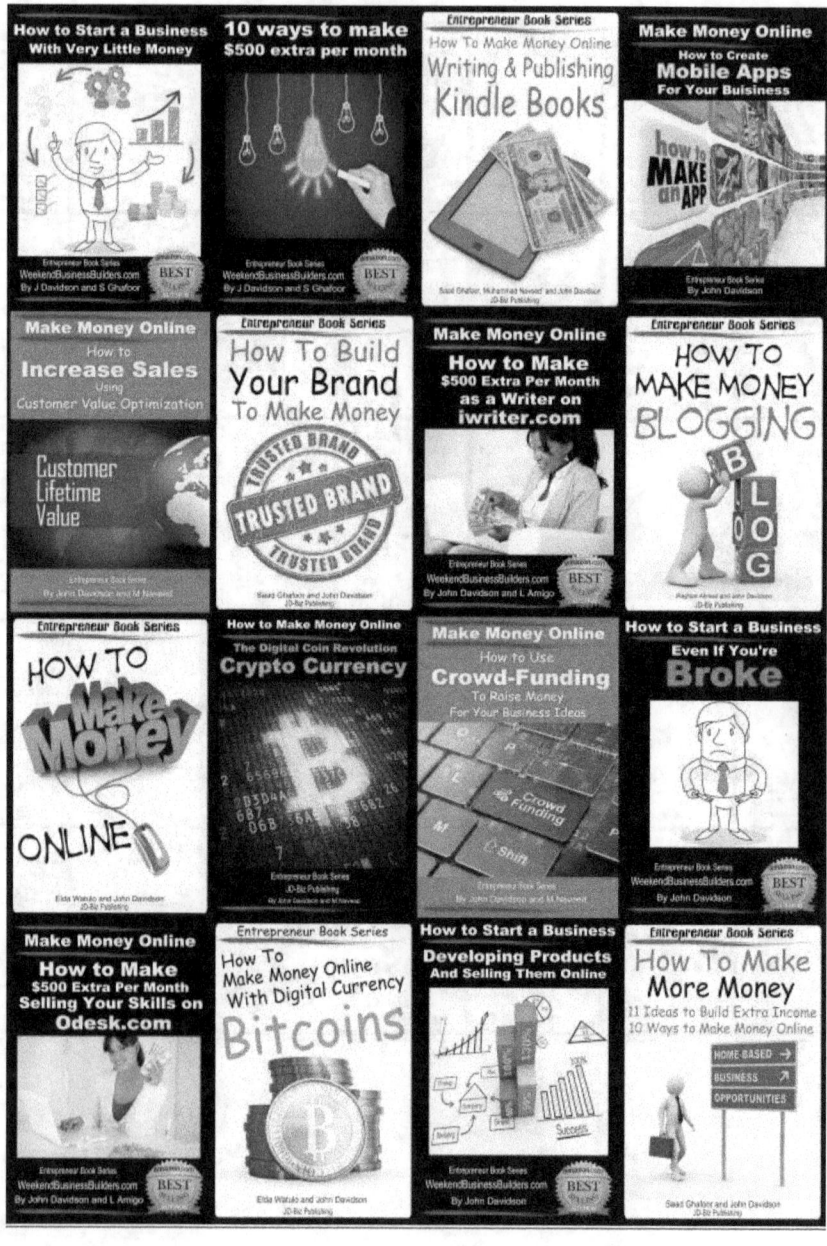

Our books are available at

1. Amazon.com

2. Barnes and Noble

3. Itunes

4. Kobo

5. Smashwords

6. Google Play Books

Publisher

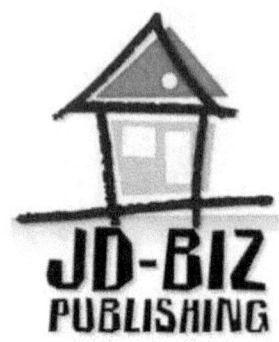

JD-Biz Corp

P O Box 374

Mendon, Utah 84325

http://www.jd-biz.com/

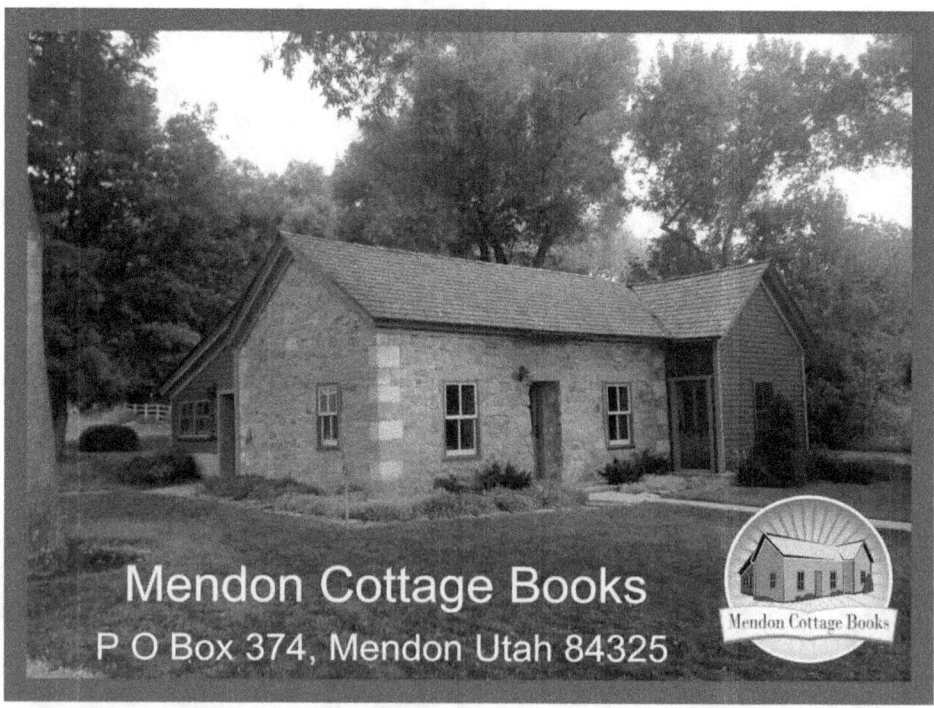

www.ingramcontent.com/pod-product-compliance
Lightning Source LLC
Chambersburg PA
CBHW070508290526
45790CB00003B/1147

* 9 7 8 1 5 1 1 5 9 2 7 6 5 *